CONTENTS

THANKS

This book would never have been written without my boyfriend's continued encouragement, Cristian Mihăilă, without his unwavering confidence in me and my ability to create a truly valuable material for people who need to lose weight. I cannot thank him enough, but I will certainly be grateful for the rest of my life.

I am extremely grateful to all my clients that I have worked with, who have trusted me to help them normalize their weight, and from which I have learned so many things. I would not be who I am today, and I could not have written this material without their contribution.

I also thank all the specialists and authors from whom I learned a lot of things, that I could then test in practice and validate. I will mention only a few of them, there are so many that I am not able to remember now.

Thousands of thanks and gratitude for: Robin Sharma, Larry Winget, Andy Szekely, Dr. Fereydoon Batmanghelidj, Dr. Eric Berg, Dr. Călin Mărginean, Prof. Dr. Gheorghe Mencinicopschi, Dr. Gabor Maté, Barbara O'Neill, Thomas deLauer, Connie Larkin.

Also thank you, the one who is reading these lines now, for your trust and the price paid for this material, and if you consider it valuable, I thank you for your contribution to promoting this book to your family, friends and acquaintances.

I hope it will be helpful for you!

INTRODUCTION

I wrote this book with all my love and joy, for those people who are willing to take responsibility for their health and life, and who are in search for those practical advices needed to reach their desired results.

I have collected and detailed in this book, 7 principles who have the biggest impact in the weight loss process, principles that I have observed and discovered in time, from my experience as a Nutritionist, with clients that I have helped to lose weight.

All the recommendations I make, are conclusions that I was able to draw on seeing the results they had or not, on my clients, depending on what they actually put into practice. Therefore, this are not theoretical and untested tips. However, even though for others worked in a certain way, it may not work for everyone in the same way and at the same pace, that is why my main recommendation is to be willing to test and experiment in your situation with patience and perseverance and find out what works best for you.

For many people in the need of losing weight, there is a need for more testing and sometimes for a longer period of time to get the desired results. I think nothing is truly universally valid, but there is certainly a set of habits suitable for each of us, we just have to discover them. In fact, it is necessary first to be willing to change, to find out what works for us, and that is actually the real challenge.

I hope from all my heart that you are not one of those, or who at least surpassed that state where you are looking for miraculous diets and ultrafast weight loss solutions. If you are in this situation, you have two choices: you can remain disappointed, because this e-book does not contain miraculous solutions, or you can choose to change, do what you have not done before and achieve the desired results.

If you choose to stay disappointed and do not put my recommendations into practice, I'm sorry for you, but you will not get your money back. I think this experience, even if you do not realize it now, helps you anyway. There will be a moment in your life when you have had enough whining and you will decide to do something meaningful with your life. So, sooner or later, I trust that you will implement the recommendations described in this book.

If you are somewhat more advanced and you are already aware that you need to learn and under-stand what you need to change to yourself and your habits, and you are willing to put it into practice in the long run, I can guarantee you that sooner or later, you will be able to reach all the weight targets that you propose.

No matter the situation you are in, I challenge you to read, re-read when you need it, then put it into practice in order to get the desired results. Simply reading these pages cannot change your life.

So be the change you want in your life, forget about excuses and trust that this time you will succeed. I trust in you!

WHY SHOULD YOU WANT TO LOSE WEIGHT WITHOUT A DIET?

In the last 5 years I have been working one to one with people who wanted to lose weight. Many of them had been before to other nutritionists or they have tried dieting, lost weight, and then put it back.

I was always asking what they expect from me, how can I help them? The most common answer was *"I want you to recommend me the best diet to lose weight quickly, what I already tried doesn't work anymore"* or *"Please tell me what to eat to lose weight, I tried to eat like the last time I lost weight, but it doesn't work anymore"*.

My approach on losing weight is **"let's learn some good habits that you can have for the rest of your life to stay in your best shape, be healthy, fit and happy"**. The people who were willing to do this became my clients and I worked with everyone until they achieved their goals or they got near it.

This sounds like a happy ending story, but the ugly truth is just beginning to unfold.

In the process, I have discovered that most of the people were not really determined to change some habits or, they were "trying" but not really doing the real work. They were coming every week with new excuses for why they can't change, because of who they can't eat healthier or what happened to them and they cannot focus on their goal anymore.

For some years I let myself fooled by their excuses, why they could not organize themselves and discipline to eat healthier, drink water, sleep, relax, learning new things and many other suggestions that I gave them. With some of them I have been working for even 1-2 years, just for small results. Yes, I have been there for them, listening to them, being supportive, reminding them that they are great people, they can do it, they deserve a better life and other things like that. I was thinking I am doing the right things, that I have to be patient with them and one day they will change.

At some point I started to feel down, to have less energy, not feeling the reward of my work, no spiritual fulfillment and also not enough money. Then I realized I was surrounded by many victims who only like to complain and they are not willing to really find a solution and do the real work on them.

I finally got a breakthrough moment and I decided to change the way I work with people, or I will end up myself being a victim, just like some of them. So, part of this change is writing this small but very comprehensive book with the most powerful advices for losing weight without crazy diets, ineffective supplements and lots of money spent meaningless.

My goal is to help you get out of the victim state, if you are there, and show you what you really need to do to solve once and for all your weight problem. If you don't feel you are a victim and you are already willing to make the real changes, good for you, you are one step forward.

So, you should learn how to lose weight without a diet because:

- It really makes you take responsibility for your whole life, to make it better;

- It forces you to find the root of the problem (why did you put this extra weight?);

- You can save time, you learn once what you have to do to stay in shape for the rest of your life, without working again and again on the same goal every year (losing weight);

- It helps you make conscious decisions regarding what you buy, eat, drink, how you sleep and many others;

- You can save lots of money spent on ineffective products that promise you to help you lose weight without too much effort (and it's not true);

- You can design your own schedule (2 meals a day, 3 meals and a snack, whatever meal schedule works for you in every moment of your life);

- You can choose what you want to eat, by listening the needs of your body.

Following a diet will not give you any of this. It will keep you asleep and you will wake up at the end of your life realizing that you have been on a diet your whole life, and for what? You didn't enjoyed the food you ate, you struggled with a rigid schedule, you didn't get to wear the clothes you liked, you didn't trust yourself enough and lived like a victim your whole life.

I don't think you want that, so, choose to change now!

BEFORE STARTING ANYTHING, FIND YOUR PURPOSE!

Finding your purpose will help you realize the root cause for depositing the extra weight. So, you need to work on eliminating the root cause, and after you achieve your weight goals, you can maintain the results for the rest of your life.

When I was asking my clients why they think they put this extra weight, they were telling me this:

- Maybe I eat too much;

- I don't have time to eat during the day and I eat too much food at dinner time;

- I like sweets and I eat lots of them every day;

- I am overweight since my childhood, I don't know why, but I want to have a normal weight now, as an adult;

- My parents are also overweight so, I think it's genes;

- I am starting to get old (like 30 years old) so I think my metabolism is getting slow;

- I think I have a slow metabolism or maybe a thyroid problem.

Those might look like some real causes, but actually, only in a few situations, eating too much at dinner and eating lots of sweets were the problems. The other reasons were never the real causes of their overweight.

Another question I have been asking my clients was *"what is your motivation, why do you want to lose weight?"*. And the most frequent answers were:

- I want to look good in the summer time (on vacation, at the beach);

- I have my wedding in a few months and I want to look good in my dress;

- I have a wedding in my family in a few months, many relatives will be there and I have to look good;

- I want to look good for my partner so he doesn't look for other women;

- I get frustrated when I go shopping, I do not find any clothes for my size;

- I don't like what I see in the mirror, I don't feel good in my skin;

- I have knee pain, back pain, it's hard to live like that, I want to get rid of the pain;

- I want to be able to play with the kids, stay healthy and live longer, for them.

Again, those might look like some real motivations, but in fact, many of them were just a surface reason.

I could see in practice that reasons like this will not get you too far. **You need to find the real reason you are willing to change**, next to this, **the real cause of your overweight** and only after that, **start working on better habits**.

I will give you a couple of examples so you can understand better what I mean.

What happens when you lie yourself

Several years ago, I had a fairly long period of time in which I experienced a series of events that I perceived to be dramatic. I thought I was a very unlucky person, that there were too many bad things happening to me, that the people around me were mean to me, that nobody understood me and did not support me, and because of that I cannot accomplish anything that I propose.

Still, I was looking for help and asking for help or at least that's what I thought I was doing.

At one point I participated in a workshop, I do not know exactly what topic, I just remember that it was supported by a lady who said she is a leader in ontological education, and through her work helps people to change their perspective on things of their life that blocks them from evolving or adversely affects their quality of life.

We were about 30 people attending that event, all women. We did various exercises together, and at one point, each of us had to choose a burning question to which we wanted to receive an answer. I still remember how preoccupied I was to look for an "intelligent" question to ask, I could not embarrass myself in front of so many women with a stupid question ... Finally, my turn comes, and I, very proud of the fact that I found a question that seemed to me to be very relevant in the context of that event, I ask: *"How can I find my motivation to do what I have to do in my business?"* At that time, I was a direct sales freelancer, I knew exactly what to do, I was intensely instructing myself to know what to do, just did not do what I knew I had to do to achieve the desired results, and when I had little success, I could not enjoy it.

The lady answered my question in a totally unexpected way for me. I do not remember the exact words, but the message was something like: "The problem is not that you have no motivation, the problem is that you are not authentic, you do not live the way you want, you do not know what you want, you did not take the time to think about it, you just struggle to do something you think you have to do or what you think people around you expect from you to do... ". I understood the value of that message only a few years later, at that moment I was too concerned about how others see me, not to see that I was drifting. I perceived this answer as a terrible humiliation, how could she have told me such a thing in front of so many women (whom I thought more "accomplished" than I, obviously), how could she break me so suddenly and harshly? I felt that now everyone "sees" how devoid of direction my life is, how helpless I feel, how vulnerable and weak...

Of course I can now share all those experiences because I no longer identify with them, I have succeeded in time to change my perception of many things and events that I have lived. I am now grateful to have found more beneficial prospects and I share my experiences whenever I have the opportunity, to provide an example for others to learn.

I know that my story is not a direct example of weight loss, but I think you understand what I wanted to convey. It does not make sense to deceive yourself with a shallow motivation, even if you manage to reach the desired weight, you will not be able to keep it in the long run.

I have seen a lot of clients who have somehow managed to use their power of will, they have tricked themselves for a while with other small rewards, and have succeeded in losing weight, but in the end, they have not achieved the state of true satisfaction and fulfillment they were expecting. Some of them manage to lose 15-20 kilograms, but they were still overweight, others showed their life partners that they could lose weight, kept weight a few months, and then started to get overweight again. I saw women who had the dream dress, the dream wedding, just a few months after, to get divorced.

It does not make sense to make such efforts!

My recommendation is to take time to discover what you really want, what's important to you, why you are really willing to make a change. Only then will you succeed in attaining the state of well-being you are looking for.

What it means to take responsibility for what you want to become

A few months ago, a young 27-year-old man, a very handsome guy, came to me to help him to lose 28 kilos. He was overweight since childhood, but he wanted to find a solution and have a normal weight. He didn't knew what a normal weight means for his age and height, but he thought that if he reaches 90 kilos he should be ok. His motivation: having no more frustrations when he goes shopping for clothes.

He had a good self-esteem and this was great, we could work on cooking, eating and sport. For the first month, I was writing for him a meal plan every week. With his food preferences, only 2 meals a day was the perfect schedule for him, at lunch eating in town and dinner, mostly cooked food by him, or a nice meal in a good restaurant, with his friends.

Meanwhile, we were also looking for the right kind of sport for him and some supplements that can really help in the process. Also he had discovered that drinking alcohol from time to time it's like a hand break for losing weight, when nothing happens for the next 3-4 days. Soon he started to sleep early and better, get up early, having more energy, more time to do what he loves.

He is a continuing learner, he read everything I recommended, he watched and listened all the video and podcasts I sent to him and many others. He understood the principles of weight loss and what living a balanced life means and he applied it in his life.

Now, he lost 22 kilos, in 14 weeks (3 months and a half) and he decided to set a new goal for 80 kilos, as a desired weight. He achieved this applying the principles I will describe you in the next chapter, but the most important, having the right mindset.

So, what he is really doing right now is:

- He is sleeping around 7-9 hours, from 23/24 in the night until 8/9 in the morning;

- He plays squash 3 times a week (60 minutes x 3);

- He takes a supplement with L-Carnitine, 3000 mg, 30 minutes before squash;

- He eats at 12-13, lunch (in a restaurant or the company cafeteria) and at 19-20, dinner (cooked by him or in a restaurant, with his friends or work colleagues);

- He drinks enough water, no coffee and no other beverages, just sometimes lemonade or maybe an alcohol free beer;

- He works 8 hours a day in a big company, at an office, but he moves from time to time (he is not stuck to his chair);

- He has his free time also, he likes biking, reading, watching or listening to educational material, on many areas of life, sometimes a cinema movie and he spends quality time with his friends;

- He is not complaining, he is supportive for his family and friends and he is an amazing example for the people around him.

I am grateful to meet and work with people like him. Everything seems so easy to do, we both have energy and it's always a pleasure to chat. I am also learning great things from him.

So you see, his real purpose is to be the person who knows he can be, to live the life he wants to live and to be an example for those around him. And he took responsibility to achieve that.

It's a proven recipe, all you need to do is to put your thought in the right order, to focus on the right things for you, to take action, and everything else will follow.

PRINCIPLES THAT HAVE THE GREATEST IMPACT ON WEIGHT LOSS

Almost every client I worked with, at first expected me to recommend less food, not to consume sugar and to exercise. They were very surprised to learn that there are many things to consider and where we have to work.

I have managed to understand this in time, only after I've noticed for a few years what, and how, it affects people, certain things that they do, or not.

From my observations, I managed to extract 7 of the

principles that have the greatest impact in the process of weight loss, and if we take them into account and put them into practice as efficiently as possible, the results are not delayed.

The seven principles are:

1. Water
2. Sleep
3. Exercise
4. Alcohol
5. The digestive system
6. Insulin
7. Dinner

I will detail each of them in the following chapters to help you understand how each principle influences the process of weight loss.

I have been trying to explain as easily as possible and understandable to all, and if you find explanations that may seem more complicated, do not worry, if you read them a few times, you will understand them.

For those of you who do not need too many details to consider these principles, at the end of each chapter you can find a short summary of what you have to do, even if you have not carefully followed all the explanations. I am glad for you, you are already a step forward, you can put more quickly into practice, and the results will show you that the principles really work.

THE FIRST PRINCIPLE – WATER

If you have been expecting for something more complicated and sophisticated, I realize that, but the most important things in life are really simple as this.

I remember my beginnings in this field, it seemed incredible for me that people come and pay me to tell them that it's good to drink water and eat some vegetables. I have been in need for some time to understand that for some people, this is a real struggle, and we all have our struggles to deal with. If this is what you need, I am here for you!

So, after oxygen, water is the next most important

thing for our body. Water is the matrix of life and there is nothing that can replace it. We can survive only 2 to 3 days without water and this shows us how important water is for our life.

I hope you don't believe that we can hydrate with liquids of any kind, because we can't. Only pure water can hydrate our cells the way our body needs. Sometimes we are told to drink a certain quantity of liquids for our health, but the message is not completely true and useful for ourselves.

How much water do we need?

Our body needs water according to many factors, so, if we are in conditions of thermal comfort, we have a normal daily activity and we are healthy, we need 30 ml of water for every kg of our body. This means that if you have 70 kilos, you need to drink 2.1 liters of water.

The true quantity that we need depends on:

- The current state of health – when we have certain conditions, we need more water;
- The temperature of the environment – when the temperature outside is high, we need more water;
- The intensity of our body activity – when we go

to gym, practice any kind of sport or we work hard, meaning when we sweat, we should drink more water;

- The intensity of our brain activity – yes, when we think harder, we need more water;

- The food we eat – when we eat something salty or we don't eat enough fruits and veggies, we should drink more water;

- The beverages we drink – when we drink alcohol or drinks with caffeine, which draws water out of the body, we need to drink more water.

Besides the quantity of water, the quality of water is also very important. We should drink a fresh water from a spring, but this kind of water is not available easily for all of us.

The best solutions are to buy a water purification system for house use, when we drink water in our home, and to buy water in glass bottles, when we want to drink water outside of our house.

A certain amount of water we can get it from our food. The best sources are fresh fruits and vegetables, but our body can extract water from tea, smoothies, soups and other types of food with an important quantity of water.

The impact of water on weight loss

I don't think I have to convince you that water does some kind of miracle on your weight loss. If water is important for our health, of course it also has a major part in weight loss. Also you should know:

- When the central control system from our brain detects low levels of energy for his functions, he generates the feelings of thirsty and hunger simultaneously. This means that we can confuse the two feelings, we don't really know if we need to drink water or to eat, and we usually go and eat. So, if we drink enough water between the meals and at least a glass of water with 30 minutes before a meal, we will be able to prevent eating too much;

- When we stress ourselves, the body starts to dehydrate, the brain needs more energy and usually we go and eat. If we drink enough water, the brain will get some energy from water and we can again prevent eating too much;

- It's very important to drink water first thing in the morning, after we wake up. Drinking 1-2 glasses of water will hydrate the body after a long night and will help eliminate the morning bowl and prevent constipation;

- It's also important to drink water before we go to sleep, with 60-90 minutes before, so we don't get up to often during the night to go to the toilet.

There are many complicated explanations why water is important on weight loss, but I don't think you need a chemistry-anatomy-biology course to understand this.

When working with people, I could really see that in those days with less water, even though they were doing everything else right, they lost less weight or even stagnated.

Short summary:

- Get used to drinking at least 30 ml of water a day, multiplied by the number of kilos you have now;
- Get used to drinking enough water in the morning after you wake up, between meals and in the evening, before bed;
- When you feel stressed, tired or hungry, first drink 1-2 glasses of water, then see if you need to eat.

THE SECOND PRINCIPLE – SLEEP

I think most people are already saying:

"sleeping is for lazy people", "we don't need to much sleep", "we are business men, we have important things to do", "time is money, we don't waste time sleeping", and other things like that.

I remember one of my clients coming one day to my office, very curious to see on the scale what his numbers are, after two weeks in which "he behaved". I was curious too because I knew him, we were struggling with some kilos for several months, and nothing happened. Every two weeks I was praying in my mind *"please God, let it be less kilos on the scale"*, but not a chance, he always came with the same weight. I thought I would lose my mind.

What the hell is happening? I know what he eats and it's ok (I asked him to send me pictures of his meals). He was a runner and he was running 3 days a week, 2 hours (he had an app and I could check on him).

I know he was drinking enough water (don't ask me how I know that, because I don't, I just believed him). I had been winning the fight with alcohol, he understood that he needs a break during this process of weight loss. And still, we were missing something.

He looked a little bit tired (of course, our meetings were always at 7:30-8 o'clock in the morning because he said he is a morning person, like me) and I asked him how many hours did he sleep. As usual, just 4-5 hours. We were negotiating for a few weeks how many hours he should sleep, but he was still "winning", meaning he didn't want to sleep more than that.

Again, I started the lecture about sleeping, how important is for weight loss, bla, bla, bla, for I don't know how many times. Because he could not bear it anymore, he said *"you know what? I don't want to sleep more, I believe sleeping is training for death"*. Then ...crickets, my brain stopped for a few seconds. What did he said? I have to write this down and analyze it. I never thought about it. Wow, what a strong belief that sleep is something bad. No wonder he did not want to sleep. With such a belief, I certainly would not have wanted to sleep either.

I have to admit that I have not succeeded in changing this belief. I have tried to explain to him in many ways, but he still believed that he is wasting time sleeping. He loves his life and he wants to live it as much as he can.

He doesn't want to sleep more than 4-5 hours a night and if this is stopping him from losing the last kilos, then that's it, he will keep the extra weight.

We don't work together anymore, but I still think about him, I wonder what he is doing. I think I will always remember him with his sleep belief, although, I hope he will change it one day and achieve the weight that he wants.

As I was saying at the beginning of this book, what we believe about something will wake up inside us some feelings, and those feeling will determine our actions towards our goals or not.

So, if you feel you have a limited belief about sleep, I hope for you that you are willing to change it. You can do it by yourself, or with the help of a therapist.

If we do not sleep enough, we can have many short-

comings, for example:

- We cannot be very productive, we think slower, we move slower, we learn slower, we solve problems slower;
- On the long term, this is how the burnout syndrome can appear;
- The regenerations and healing function does not work efficiently;
- The risk of developing type 2 diabetes increases;
- The risk of obesity increases.

And those are just a few examples, but the damage can be even bigger.

Studies show that the average American is sleeping only 6 hours and 51 minutes per night.

Top performers, like athletes, public speakers, successful business people, get 8 hours and 36 minutes of sleep a night.

To lose weight, we need at least 7 and a half hours of sleep per night and even more.

Now, to sleep enough and effective, you need to do a few things:

- Stop any light and screen activity with 1 hour before bed, meaning no telephone, no TV, no laptop, Kindle and any other devices like that. You need to let the body produce the sleep hormone, melatonin, so you can be able to fall asleep;

- You should fall asleep with as many hours as you can before midnight, it would be ideal around 22;

- You need to stop drinking coffee at latest 2 PM, coffee will still be in your system for the next 6 hours and if you keep drinking later than 2 PM, you can have trouble falling asleep;

- You need to drink water before bed, but with 60-90 minutes before falling asleep, so you don't wake up during the night and go to the toilet;

- Take you dinner with at least 3-4 hours before bed and a lightly dinner, food easy to digest;

- Don't take pills to help you fall asleep, you better solve the real problem with insomnia, maybe you worry too much, you are depressive, or you just don't try the things above, simple things, but very effective.

Short summary:

- To lose weight effectively, you need to sleep at least 7 and a half hours a night;
- Try to sleep as much as possible 1-2 hours before midnight;

- Get used to stopping any bright screen at least 1 hour before your sleep.

THE THIRD PRINCIPLE – EXERCISE

This is one of my favorite subjects to talk about. There are a lot of myths about physical exercises for weight loss and there are many battles between nutritionists and personal trainers about this topic.

Nutritionists claim that when you want to lose weight, 80% it's about food, and only 20% about exercises and the personal trainers claim that if you do not workout, you have no chance to lose weight or that it's not healthy to lose weight without workout.

Of course the truth is somewhere in between and I can tell you, from practice with lots of clients, how things work.

I have to tell you that most of my clients came to me because they didn't like to workout and they wanted to lose weight without being forced to move in any way. I tried to convince them that physical exercise is good for the health, not only for weight loss, but again I have to admit I did not succeed to do that. However, at least I can tell how things have been working out for them.

All the clients that have been eating the right food, drinking enough water, sleeping, but didn't practice any kind of physical exercise, at some point, they stopped losing weight, although they needed to still lose some important amount of kilos. Yes, they could lose from 12 kilos and even up to 22 kilos without exercise, but they failed to lose the total number of kilos they wanted. So, this means that those clients, they could not achieve the final goal, they stopped long before that. More than that, on long term, meaning even 2 to 3 years, even they kept eating healthy, they maintained the weight, but they did not lose that final extra weight.

Now, let me tell you about the few clients that were willing to find the right exercise for them and to include it in their lifestyle. Those people, even after we stopped working together, they kept losing weight, they achieved the final goal and sometimes even more.

From my perspective, we should move the body because it's a natural thing, we were not created to stay on a chair or a couch all day long. We need to move as much as we can!

Now, I want to give you just a few benefits to move your body:

- Physical movement builds muscle mass and prevents muscle breakdown, to be used like fuel;

- Physical movement stimulates the activity of burning enzymes to produce the energy required for muscle activity;

- Physical activity burns some amino acids as fuel, so that it does not reach toxic levels in our bodies;

- Physical activity prevents high blood pressure;

- Physical movement lowers blood glucose levels in diabetics and reduces the need for insulin;

- Physical movement determine the liver to produce glucose from the fat it has as a deposit or the fat from the blood;

- Physical activity strengthens the bones of the body and helps prevent osteoporosis;

- Physical activity increases the production of vital

hormones, improves libido and increases sexual performance;

- Physical movement stimulates the production of endorphins, the natural sedatives of the body that give the same sense of euphoria that drug addiction is trying to achieve through abusive consumption.

Of course that are many more benefits in moving the body, I only gave you a few and mostly the ones who are related with weight loss and a good well-being.

Which are the best forms of physical activity?

The best form of physical activity that we can benefit from in the long run, without damaging the joints, is ... (drum sound) WALKING.

Now, don't tell me it's too simple and too good to be true. Yes, it's simple and it's true, it works. Walking is the most natural body movement that we can do. It's also free and easy to do it, if you want to...

An hour of walking activates enzymes that burn fat, enzymes that remain active for 12 hours. So, one morning and one evening walk will keep these enzymes active throughout the day and will cause cholesterol deposits in the arterial system to clear.

Other forms of physical movement beneficial to the body and with a great impact on weight loss are: swimming, golf, skiing, skating, rock climbing, tennis, squash, cycling, tai chi, danceing, aerobic movement.

Exercises in the open air are even more beneficial than those practiced indoors. Thus, our body connects better with nature.

So, I encourage you to find the most suitable form of physical activity for you, to include it in your lifestyle and to enjoy a long and beautiful life.

Short summary:

- You should include physical exercise in your lifestyle for both health benefits and weight loss benefits;
- The simplest and most natural form of physical activity is WALKING;
- Exercise releases into the body endorphins, substances that give a good feeling in the body, as well as hugs, chocolate and sex.

THE FOURTH PRINCIPLE – ALCOHOL

We all know that alcohol does not contain essential nutrients and we do not need it in our diet, but many people are consuming it without realizing the great disadvantages it brings, especially when we talk about weight loss.

As far as I noticed, most people think alcohol should be avoided in the weight loss process because it has many calories, and those who are concerned to keep a significant caloric deficit for weight loss, realize that there is no place for alcohol.

It is true that alcohol has many calories. It's somewhere between proteins, carbohydrates and fats. Proteins and carbohydrates have 4 calories per gram, fats have 9 calories per gram, and alcohol has 7 calories per gram. However, not only the number of calories is the disadvantage.

The main drawbacks and barriers that alcohol brings to the weight loss process:

- Alcohol is a toxin for the liver, and for this reason, when alcohol enters the body, the liver takes care as a priority of his metabolism, putting on hold a number of other processes, including the burning of fat. The fat burning process is delayed with 48 to 72 hours, so in this time you do not lose weight;

- Alcohol, although it has calories, does not give the body its satiety, because it does not contain the nutrients the body needs. Moreover, it even increases the appetite and increases the risk of eating excessively while drinking alcohol;

- Alcohol consumption disrupts the senses, reduces will power, and this leads to decreased awareness of the quantity of food eaten and the quantity of alcohol consumed;

- Regularly consumed alcohol prevents the natural regeneration of the liver that affects both the process of weight loss, as well as many other important processes in the body.

I don't want to insist too much on the drawbacks of drinking alcohol, we all know that it is a drug that produces addiction and that it would be good to consume it in moderation. Although I personally rarely drink alcohol, I do not claim that we shouldn't consume at all, I just want to point out that in the process of weight loss, alcohol has the same effect as the handbrake to the car when the car is driven, the car doesn`t move. So the alcohol puts a stop to weight loss process for a long period of time, especially if it is consumed constantly.

Now, the good news is that alcohol may be consumed in moderation in the weight-loss process, without slowing down the process, as follows:

- Instead of consuming the amount of alcohol you want for a few days in a row, better choose a day when you drink alcohol, then leave a long rest period; for example, you can consume alcohol on a Friday or Saturday night, then take a break of at least two weeks and even more, depending on how quickly you want to lose weight;

- Take a food supplement containing the B complex after drinking alcohol to help restore the liver faster and avoid hangover;

- Eat less fat and meals with a high percentage of fibers the day you consume alcohol;

- Make sure you hydrate yourself very well during the day you drink alcohol and the next day, both for your health and for avoiding the hangover the next day.

Regarding the type of alcoholic beverage consumed, it would be preferable consuming alcoholic beverages containing the smallest amount of carbohydrates. Thus, it would be preferable to have stronger drinks, to the detriment of wine, beer and very sweet alcoholic beverages. Also, you should avoid mixed drinks, such as cocktails, because they contain a lot of calories.

I know that alcohol, as well as food, is very much associated with well-being, socialization, sometimes even with reward, and for some people it has become the way they can cope with the challenges of life. I do not want to take the joy of socializing and feeling good, I just want to remind you to be careful not to make excesses, but to keep a moderation that will only bring you benefits, not disadvantages.

I had the opportunity to see how many customers, both women and men, consistently sabotaged their alcohol consumption outcomes for many reasons. I hope that you, the one who reads these lines, become more aware of the impact of alcohol in the weight loss process, and if you do not think so, experiment and you will notice the results on your body.

Short summary:

- When the liver detects the presence of alcohol in the body, it treats it with priority, and fat burning is stopped and postponed for up to 72 hours;
- Alcohol has no nutritional value and no real benefit for the body, but it can bring many disadvantages, so consume it with moderation;
- When drinking alcohol, drink plenty of water at the same time, eat high fiber and low fat meals.

THE FIFTH PRINCIPLE – DIGESTIVE SYSTEM

Do not be scared, I will not teach you a detailed anatomy course at this point, but I will very simply explain the role that the digestive system has in the weight loss process and what to do to make sure it works best.

I noticed that most people think eating is equal to feeding us. We fill our dishes with something that seems to be food, we swallow it somehow, until it seems to us that we are full, and sometimes even more, after which we are comfortable; that`s it, we have done our job, next the body knows how to digest and absorb nutrients. In reality, I think we have some more responsibility, but do not realize it. We need to make sure we did the right thing so that the body can make an optimal digestion and absorb the nutrients. I think it is the duty of each of us to know our body to a certain extent, to know how it works and what we have to do to be healthy and to have a wellbeing throughout the life.

The digestive system is an ensemble of organs that digests and absorbs ingested foods as well as evacuating unassimilable residues.

The digestive system consists of:

1. Digestive tube - a series of tubular organs of different sizes:

- The oral cavity (tongue and teeth);

- Pharynx (the connection between the oral cavity and the esophagus);

- Esophagus (makes the connection between pharynx and stomach);

- The stomach (the most dilated segment of the digestive tract);

- Intestine (the longest segment of the digestive tract, here up to 90% of nutrients are absorbed);

- Large intestine (here are absorbed non-assimilated nutrients from the small intestine, and unassimilable residues are eliminated).

2. Accessory organs - at different stages of the digestive tract:

- Salivary glands (secretes saliva, and the digestive process is triggered in the mouth);

- Liver (releases the bile, a necessary secretion in the digestion process);

- Pancreas (releases pancreatic juice, a liquid capable of degrading all types of food).

The main function of the digestive system is to prepare the food needed for the cells of the body, and this process is done by digestion and absorption.

Please stay with me and keep reading, I promise that things start to become interesting.

We need to know briefly what the digestive system is, to understand what digestion is and how important it is to have optimal digestion. What does optimal digestion mean? A process that unfolds normally and after which the body can absorb the necessary nutrients.

Digestion starts in the oral cavity and for this reason, it is very important that we chew well enough the foods we want to eat. Further, the stomach will continue the process of physical food grinding, a process started in the oral cavity, where, if we did not chew well enough, we practically give it more work to the stomach and we are beginning to make it harder to digest.

Gastric digestion occurs in the stomach where the alimentary bolus is broken down by gastric juice and enzymes from the stomach through tonic movements, adaptive and peristaltic movements of the stomach muscles. Further, depending on the type of food consumed and the intensity of peristaltic movements of the stomach, depends the process of emptying the stomach.

After being processed in the stomach, food passes into the small intestine, and most of the digestion takes place here. At this level, three fluids are released for digestion: the bile (produced by the liver), the pancreas juice (produced by the pancreas) and the intestinal juice (produced by the intestinal glands). These digestive juices are alkaline, and the pH level is high in the small intestine. This creates an environment conducive to molecular degradation, which allows the absorption of nutrients through the intestinal wall into the blood that reaches the liver, where filtration, detoxification and nutrient processing takes place.

Further, through peristaltic movements, oscillation, periodic contracting, food mass reaches the large intestine. Here, depending on the type of food consumed, the food meal is retained enough time to allow fermentation and decompose, to break down unprocessed elements in the small intestine. After the absorption of the last nutrients takes place, the waste is stored for a while, and through peristaltic movements are to be evacuated.

The correct development of all these processes has a major impact primarily on general health, but also on the weight loss process. When the body does not receive the necessary nutrients, due to inappropriate digestion, it will not easily consume the adipose tissue reserves, and even more, it will tend to store it further.

Another problem that may occur and slows the weight loss process is constipation, the body eliminates to late the waste it no longer needs.

The good news is that we can implement a few habits that help us maintain a healthy digestive system and lose weight:

- Since digestion starts from the mouth, it is important to chew well the foods we eat;

- It is important to drink plenty of water during the day, but not during meals, in order not to dilute the gastric juices and the digestion process in the stomach. Of course, no other beverages should be drunk during meals, except for herbal teas, which can be consumed unsweetened during meals, sometimes;

- It is important to learn not to combine too much food at a table because digestion will be difficult (for example, it would be better not to combine meat and potatoes or cereals, not to consume all kinds of animal protein at the same meal, not to combine foods containing starch with fermented foods, etc.);

- Regular exercise helps both in maintaining overall health, but contributes significantly to the digestion process by increasing the intensity of peristaltic movements in the digestive tract;

- Constipation can be avoided with effective hydration, eating foods with high fiber concentration (vegetables, nuts, seeds, fruits, legumes, whole grains) and exercise.

I tried to explain you as simply as possible the importance of optimal functioning of the digestive system, and if it still seems complicated, I encourage you to take the time to read and to have patience until you finally understand your body and your responsibility, learn how it works and what you need to do to keep it healthy.

If you need and want to find out what foods and combinations of foods are easy to digest, don`t worry, you will find it in Chapter 7, just keep reading.

Short summary:

- Digestion starts from inside the mouth, food should be chewed well enough before it gets into the stomach;
- It is important to have an optimal digestion in order to efficiently absorb the nutrients from the diet and the body to easily allow burning of the fat deposits;
- Exercise plays an important role in effective intestinal transit and constipation prevention.

THE SIXTH PRINCIPLE – INSULIN

Most of the time, when talking about insulin, we only do it in the circumstances where we talk about diabetes, we rarely think about the role it has in fattening and implicitly in weight loss. And when we talk about fattening and weight loss, we think about "what" we did when we got fat or "what" to do to lose weight. I think a better question would be "why?". Why does the body get fat?

Fattening is only a symptom of a body that is no longer so healthy and sometimes very sick. We did not take care to provide the necessary conditions for a good functioning, we took it for granted, and just exploited it without taking responsibility for taking care of it. Yes, our body is a very intelligent and a complex system capable of self-regulation, but it also depends to a certain extent on our contribution, beneficial or less beneficial.

Weight loss is a consequence of beneficial actions on the body. A body that gets better, will self-adjust itself. If it needs to heal, it will heal, if it needs to lose weight, it will lose weight.

Insulin is the hormone that prevents us from losing weight. Even in the presence of a small amount of insulin in the body, all fat burning processes are stopped.

Insulin is a hormone produced by the pancreas. It`s role is to direct blood glucose (which forms after each meal) inside all the cells that need energy. It works as a key that opens the door to the inside of the cells for the intake of glucose. When the amount of glucose in the blood is much higher than the energy requirement of the cells, insulin stores excess glucose in the first phase in the form of glycogen (a short-term energy reserve in the liver and muscle, quickly accessible), and second phase, in the form of adipose tissue (a long-term energy reserve, much more difficult to access).

The real problem occurs when the body develops a pre-diabetic disorder called insulin resistance. Although the pancreas produces insulin, it is not recognized at the cellular level (the key does not open the door), and glucose remains in the blood in large quantities. In an attempt to normalize the blood glucose level, the pancreas will produce even more insulin, and this will lead to dyslipidemia (high blood triglycerides, high "bad" cholesterol and low "good" cholesterol), type 2 diabetes, increased blood pressure and obesity.

After a time when "the pancreas sees" that even increased insulin production does not solve the situation, it may end up producing no insulin at all, and this is the type 1 diabetes in which people have to inject their insulin from outside.

Now don`t be sad, it is a long way to this unwanted stage, that is only after many years of unhealthy habits you arrive here, not overnight. So let's see what we have to do to maintain the proper functioning of our body.

In the weight loss process, a major goal should be to maintain a low level of insulin as possible, of course, at the same time a normal level of blood glucose.

So here are some habits that we can implement to achieve this:

1. Glucose increases in blood automatically after each meal and inevitably a certain amount of insulin will be released, but depending on what we eat and the number of daily meals, the amount of insulin you need may be higher or lower. To keep a low amount of insulin, we have some solutions:

- The number of daily meals should not be very high, it would be ideal to eat only 2-3 meals (2 main meals, 2 main meals and a snack or even 3 main meals). Overly frequent meals and "snaking" continue throughout the day can permanently maintain insulin in the blood, almost blocking the weight loss process;

- Each food has a glycemic index, it measures the intestinal absorption rate, meaning the rate at which glucose reaches the blood. The higher this speed, the faster and in a higher amount, insulin will be released. So when we want to lose weight, it's more important to follow the glycemic index of foods, more than the calories count. We do not need to completely eliminate carbohydrate in the diet, but we can choose to consume those foods that have a medium and low glycemic index, and those with a high glycemic index, eat them in smaller quantities:

o High glycemic index means between 110 and 55 (e.g.: beer 110, dextrose 100, fries 95, gluten-free white bread 90, corn flakes 85, potato 80, croissant / sugar 70, juices 70, bread of whole grains / muesli 65, pizza 60, ketchup 55, etc.);

o An average glycemic index is between 50 and 40 (e.g.: mango / sweet potatoes 50, peas / tomato sauce 45, oats / sugar-free peanut butter 40, etc.);

o Small glycemic index means between 35 and 5 (e.g.: black beans / wild rice / apples / oranges / plums / sunflower / sesame seeds 35, raw carrot / dark lentils / garlic / tomatoes /grapefruit / pomelo / pears / apricots 30, berries / strawberries / cherries / green lentils / humus / black chocolate 25, lemon / cocoa powder / soy yogurt without flavorings 20, broccoli / cauliflower / mushrooms / green lettuce / spinach / tofu / almonds 15, avocado 10, shellfish / vinegar / spices 5).

2. Physical exercise contributes to the normalization of blood glucose and causes the body to access long-term energy deposits, adipose tissue;

3. Intermittent fasting - alternating feeding intervals with fasting, as well as physical exercise, allow the body to access fat stores for energy production in the absence of insulin due to longer periods of time where food is not consumed. A very practical form of intermittent fasting is 8/16 (2-3 meals may be consumed within 8 hours, followed by a 16-hour period when no food and beverages containing calories are consumed, only water and possibly tea or unsweetened coffee);

I think you've already started to understand better the impact of our daily habits on weight loss. We need to pay attention to many aspects than the food itself, when we have the goal of weight loss. For this reason, just following a simple diet will not be enough for weight loss, it`s only on a short-term.

Short summary:

- When the body releases insulin in the blood, fat burning is stopped;
- To keep insulin as low as possible, too frequent meals should be avoided, and foods consumed should be in the category of those with a low and medium glycemic index;
- Exercise and intermittent fasting also help maintain low insulin levels.

THE SEVENTH PRINCIPLE – DINNER

"Finally, we're talking about food", some of those who have come to read to this point will say. Yes, we also talk about food and of course it is important and what we actually eat to lose weight, but it was important to first understand how the digestive system works and the role of insulin, so that you can finally understand the impact of the food in weight loss.

Most diets are developed around a major impact principle, but taken and treated in isolation, such as:

- High protein diets (Atkins, Dukan) - gives you great results in weight loss and seem to be easy to put into practice because foods high in carbohydrates and high glycemic index are eliminated, so, it only remains those foods that do not trigger insulin, satiety due to protein consumption it is satisfactory and does not allow excess food to be consumed, so there are enough meals with few calories, but it does not take too much into account the importance of rapid digestion, the harmful effects of excess protein consumption and does not promote sport next to the diet;

- Dissociated diets - gives you results because the principle of optimal digestion is respected by eating separate foods on a group basis (in one day meat, in one day dairy products, in one day carbohydrates, in one day fruits and vegetables, or several food combinations that still allow easy digestion and fast). The problem is that it does not have a continuity, it can`t be transformed into a lifestyle that allows weight maintenance, and the body, after it returns to its initial eating habits, so are the kilos;

- Ketogenic diet (high fat diet recommended) - This diet takes into account the role of insulin in the body, promotes the consumption of foods with low glycemic index, which keep blood glucose under control, the degree of satiety is high and offers comfort, allows easy alleviation and even alleviation of many affections. It can be introduced into our lifestyle, but it requires a lot of discipline to eat exactly the necessary proportions of fat, protein and carbohydrates. For this reason, many people are basically just trying to keep this diet, but they actually do a lot of mistakes, and there are no benefits, and more, they can have many disadvantages;

- The Paleolithic diet (the diet our ancestors had prior to the development of agriculture and grain crops on a large scale) - a very low consumption of cereals and vegetables is practiced, and in this way, the principle of optimal digestion is respected and the importance of insulin. It can easily lose weight, the degree of satiety is big enough and can be introduced into lifestyle, and alongside all other principles, can maintain a normal weight and good health throughout life.

From my point of view, the ideal diet should be set for each one of us, and it would be the sum of principles and rules that make sense and we feel it is right for each and one of us.

But in order to do this, we need first to find out some information, then to put it into practice and to find out what works and what`s not for each of us and finally to draw our own conclusions.

Turning to food and dining, as I have already said, the daily number of meals we should have is somewhere around 2-3 meals. Of course, it is important to eat nutritious foods, all the meals to be as balanced as possible and to keep as close as possible the amount of calories needed for our daily consumption without excess.

However, in the times we live, maintaining a perfect balance between all this can be quite challenging. For this reason, when we talk about weight loss, the biggest impact on the weight loss process has the dinner. Although it is important to eat throughout the day, what we eat in the evening may cause to a greater extent whether we lose weight or not.

Our body, whether we like it or not, whether we believe it or not, works at a natural rhythm that we cannot change according to our will. In the morning when waking up, after the sun rises, our body wakes up and prepares for action. Both for day-to-day actions and for its internal processes, which we may not sometimes realize, the body needs fuel, nutrients. Even when we sit for a whole day in the home and maybe even in bed without much physical effort, our body needs a certain amount of fuel, a certain amount of calories introduced into the system, so it can work correct, what is called basic metabolism. Besides this minimum amount of calories, depending on the daily effort, our body needs to receive a number of additional calories, but not calories of any kind, but calories that contain the necessary nutrients.

A man who has a normal weight, who does not need to lose weight, basically before starting the day's actions, should begin to fuel himself, that is to take what is called breakfast, a meal that it would bring the fuel required for operation for several hours. The next meal should be lunch, which will fuel it until the evening. A person who finishes most of his daily activities sometime around 18 o'clock may have dinner somewhere around 19 o'clock and at this meal it would be sufficient to consume a fairly small amount of easily digestible food that would help the body during the night in reconstruction processes during sleep.

People who manage to have such a program are people who maintain a good health and a normal weight.

Unfortunately, not all people on the planet manage to keep this balance, and from what we can see, many of them needs to learn how to reach this balance.

But first, let's see how people get extra weight. Simply enough by:

- A first cause is dehydration, and instead of drinking more water, people get to eat more food;
- For various reasons, they do not sleep enough, and

usually the evening meal is taken very late and is too abundant;

- They have a sedentary lifestyle, they do not move their body well enough at a natural pace, but spend a lot of time in the car, on the chair and even on the couch;

- They consume alcohol with too much frequency, and many of them daily;

- They have the habit of combining food in an inappropriate way or prefer food dishes that are very tasty, but made from totally inappropriate combinations of ingredients, which greatly hinder digestion and favors fat deposit;

- They consume too much foods with high glycemic index (cereals, sugar, products containing artificial substances, excess fruits, excess sweets, juices), they have too many daily meals and even they snack throughout the day;

- They consume too much food and hardly digestible combinations at the evening meal (fast food, meat with rice or potatoes and bread, pizza, meat pasta or fatty cheese pasta, meat pies or cheese pie, fat-rich cheeses, sweets and fruit after dinner or even instead of dinner, etc.).

Evening meals for people who need to lose weight, but also for those who want to maintain a normal body weight and good health, should be made up of choices such as:

- Fish or seafood cooked with a low fat or non-fat addition, on the grill or in the oven, with cooked vegetables aside (vegetables such as asparagus, broccoli, cauliflower, Brussels sprouts, carrots, sweet potatoes, pumpkins, onions, celery, artichokes, green beans, but not potatoes) and a green lettuce salad (baby spinach, arugula, kale, iceberg salad, Roman lettuce and any other salad, olive oil and a little balsamic vinegar or lemon);

- A vegetable soup with or without meat, but without croutons or any bread (even soups containing a little meat are good because they contain a very small quantity and it is cooked, and the whole meal will have fewer calories);

- A salad with green leaves (kale, baby spinach, arugula, any other type of salad), raw vegetables (tomatoes, cucumbers, peppers, radishes, onions, apio celery, fennel, raw carrot, any other kind of raw vegetables will like), a source of vegetable fats (avocados, olives, nuts, seeds, olive oil) and a protein source (beef / pork / poultry, fish or seafood, or chickpeas / lentils / quinoa for vegans);

- From time to time, a roast of lean meats can also be served with cooked vegetables and lettuce aside, but not very often because the meat is digested in a longer period of time and is likely to make it harder to sleep (holding the body busy with digestion);

- It would be ideal to avoid the dairy products that are hardest to digest in the evening, especially fatty dairy products (French cheese, halloumi cheese, gourmet mozzarella and many more);

- Also, the evening meal should be low in carbohydrates (we will not have time to consume so much energy as we prepare for sleep);

- After dinner don't eat dessert or fruits;

- It would be ideal to take the evening meal 3-4 hours before sleep, which in turn should be before midnight.

In the evening our body prepares for sleep, and all metabolic processes are getting slower. As a result, if we have a rich meal, digestion will take place too slowly, we will not rest properly and excess calories will be stored in the form of fat.

Short summary:

- While it is important to eat throughout the day, what we eat at dinner determines to the greatest extent whether we lose weight or not;
- Dinner should be easily digestible and taken 3-4 hours before sleep;
- After dinner, it would be better not to eat any fruit or sweets.

So, in the end, I will recall the seven principles that have the greatest impact on the weight loss process:

-        Hydrate yourself efficiently every day, water is vital and it's so easy to consume;

-        Sleep well and be careful to have a restful sleep, there is no substitute for this principle and its benefits;

-        Move your body as naturally as you like, don't torture yourself by practicing sports that you do not like;

-        Consume alcohol in moderation, and during weight loss, it would be best if you take a break, to not slow down the process too much;

-        Eat especially easily digestible foods and combinations of foods that are easily decomposed and absorbed by the body;

-        Keep insulin under control by eating foods with low glycemic index and a small number of meals, and to whom it fits as a meal schedule, intermittent fasting comes with countless benefits;

-        Always eat an easy meal to digest, nourishing, and with as few calories as possible.

FINAL CONCLUSIONS

I've been looking to give you the most valuable information I have accumulated over my experience as a nutritionist, and I hope I've been able to pass it on in a simple and easy way to understand.

Even if you have come to the end of this book, in fact, your work is just starting now. Simply reading this book, without implementing the principles described, will not bring you any benefit or result.

Certainly many things you already know or heard, but you have not put them into practice so far. I wish from all my heart that this time you can implement them, because that is how you can get results.

If you do not like what you found out of this book or do not think these recommendations work, and you still look for miraculous diets and tips to relieve you from your personal effort to change yourself, then I can only wish you an easy suffering as possible, because that's what waits you anyway.

Nothing will change for the better in your life, if you do not consciously choose to give up excuses, suffering and chaos, be willing to change your thoughts, emotions and actions in order to reach the desired results.

I wish for you to love yourself, to be patient and indulgent with yourself, to be persevering and to achieve all the goals for your weight and health.